The LeRu Wellness Guide to Pain and Fatigue Management

Improving Symptoms associated with Chronic Fatigue, Fibromyalgia, Long Covid and More

By
Sarah Pearson

Copyright © 2024 by Sarah Pearson

All rights reserved.

No portion of this book may be reproduced in any form without written permission from the publisher or author.

This publication is designed to provide accurate and authoritative information in regard to the subject matter covered, at the time of publication. While the author has used their best efforts in preparing this book, they make no representations or warranties with respect to the accuracy or completeness of the contents of this book. The advice and strategies contained herein may not be suitable for your situation and is for information purposes. It does not replace medical advice. You should consult with a health professional when appropriate. Neither the publisher nor the author shall be liable for any loss of profit or any other commercial damages, including but not limited to special, incidental, consequential, personal, or other damages.

Book Cover by Get Covers

ISBN: 978-1-0686211-0-9

Also available from the same author:

The LeRu Wellness Guide to Sleep

www.leru-wellness.co.uk

Contents

Hi and Welcome...7

Introduction..9

Know your Triggers...19

Exercise..21

Looking after your Mental Health......................................31

Cryo- and Heat Therapy...43

Nutrition..47

Complementary Therapies...61

Essential Oils..69

Your 'Bad Day' Toolkit...83

Over to You..87

Essential Oil usage and Safety Advice............................101

Thank You..106

Resources..108

www.leru-wellness.co.uk

Hi and Welcome!

My name is Sarah Pearson and I've been a Complementary Therapist for over fifteen years. I trained as a therapist in 2006, after a Reflexology session changed my life. I'd been struck with a 'mystery illness' which had left doctors baffled. Several tests and a stay in hospital with no answers left them to conclude I had Chronic Fatigue, no treatment was available and I was to get on with my life. Barely able to walk and housebound for months, a chance recommendation led me to give Reflexology a try. For the first time in months not only could I walk again, but the brain-fog lifted, the headaches ceased and my appetite returned. It felt nothing short of a miracle!

Of course if you're reading this, I assume you also have some kind of chronic health issue and will know that the road to recovery is never that straight forward. There were setbacks, there have been many symptoms I've learnt to live with and have become my 'normal'. This last year has seen me struggle with similar issues and I'm currently trapped in the system of tests, NHS waiting lists and Doctors who don't seem to be listening.

I'm telling you my story because I want you to know I truly understand how you feel. I know what it is like to wake up each day not knowing if you have the energy to even get dressed, when every movement is like wading through treacle and you cannot concentrate enough to even hold a basic conversation. In this book you are going to be challenged, I'm going to make you reflect and ask questions you may not like, I'm going to give you some tough-love. But please believe me when I say that I am not trying to patronise you or that I don't understand what you are going through. I am doing it *because* I understand what you are going through.

Over the years I've treated hundreds maybe even into the thousand clients with chronic pain and fatigue related conditions such as; Fibromyalgia, Chronic Fatigue, Autoimmune conditions, Arthritis and more recently Long Covid. This guide is a culmination of my research, training and experience of working with such clients.

Introduction

Pain and Fatigue are common symptoms which can have multiple causes. In my experience as a massage therapist, they are the two symptoms I see the most of and the two often appear together. In terms of holistic health, they both have similar treatments, hence me covering both in the one book.

I cannot stress enough how important it is to see your GP in the first instance of pain and fatigue symptoms. More than likely a simple blood test will show something which can be easily treated e.g. low iron or thyroid issues. It may show further tests are needed, if so again hopefully you will receive treatment.

There are however, several conditions which will not show any abnormalities on blood tests and for which, mainstream medicine struggles to treat. These conditions include but are not limited to; Fibromyalgia, Chronic Fatigue, Autoimmune conditions, Arthritis and more recently Long Covid. This book is intended to be a guide for such conditions.

www.leru-wellness.co.uk

I make no claim that you will be 'cured', in fact I'm quite sceptical of such claims. If you see so called 'healers' claiming that they can cure you with a single supplement, product or treatment, then run and certainly do not part with your money! True healing is not found in a single treatment. It is often seeing small improvements from a variety of methods which cumulates over time. What we are more likely seeing with these 'miracles' is someone going into remission I.e. they have discovered a way which works for them, to keep their symptoms manageable, but without a concerted effort, their condition is likely to return. When dealing with chronic conditions, remission is exactly what we are aiming to achieve.

We all respond differently to treatments, whether a conventional treatment or not (this is why some people can get side-effects to medication whilst others do not). So, just because a treatment has worked for someone else does not mean it will work for you. Unfortunately this means you may need to try a myriad of treatments before you find one which suits you. I understand how frustrating (and expensive) this can be, but sometimes knowing what doesn't work can be just as valuable.

The road to healing is never easy. It is common to experience large improvements only to see a small decline, probably not quite back to square one and to then have this process repeat itself. Expect set backs along the way; prolonged periods of feeling 'normal' only to have random days when symptoms flare-up again.

Unfortunately for us sufferers, doctors tend to be right when they say we need to learn to live with a condition. That doesn't mean however that you will not improve. It does mean you need to prioritise your health and wellbeing, rediscover your body and it's limitations and potentially make some big changes to your lifestyle.

Let's begin by discussing pain. There are three main types of pain; acute meaning short term pain e.g. an injury which alerts us we need to stop and address the issue. This is actually a good form of pain as it makes us stop, take action and thus prevent the situation from becoming worse. The second type of pain is chronic or persistent i.e. long-term pain which affects everyday life and the third, intermittent pain is similar to chronic pain except it comes and goes. For the purposes of this book we are concerned with chronic and intermittent pain.

These types of pain don't really serve a purpose in terms of alerting us something is wrong and needs addressing. Instead, they become a frustration which reduces our mobility, impacts our sleep, increases irritability and lowers our mood. This can obviously have an effect on our work, social lives and daily living.

Pain is caused by nerves sending messages to the brain. With chronic pain, for reasons often unknown, these pain signals go haywire or into overdrive. This often results in pain where there is no physical reason, or pain seemingly in places where the origin is in another place. Arthritis is a common example of this and I witness it countless times in the treatment room too; clients will tell me they have knee or hip pain for example but the reason is sometimes high or flat foot arches. Sometimes we can address the actual origins of the pain which in turn corrects where the pain is felt. Or, more commonly, we need to calm down the nervous system i.e. those haywire pain signals, to retrain the brain that we are not in pain.

Research is ongoing in this area with regards to the Vagus Nerve. This nerve is the longest in the body and is associated with regulating digestion, heart rate, mood and receptors in the skin (for heat, touch, pain etc). Scientists believe it may have a role in conditions such as Fibromyalgia and Rheumatoid arthritis. However it is too early to draw any real conclusions but may offer hope in the future as a treatment for such conditions. Devices which stimulate the vagus nerve are currently available for people with some forms of epilepsy and severe depression, and scientists are currently researching whether the treatment is suitable for people with fibromyalgia etc. Of course, this could take years and so in the meantime, for those who wish to regulate the vagus nerve, lifestyle methods such as those described in this book are the only viable option.

The area of the brain which tells us we are in pain is close to the part of the brain which signals our emotions. If pain is felt, it will have a negative affect on the surrounding areas of the brain. This is why when we feel down, stressed or anxious our pain may feel worse. Of course this is a chicken and egg scenario, is the pain making us down or is the fact we are down causing the pain? It is unfortunately the reason why many sufferers do not feel believed over their pain with claims it is 'in the mind' or they are imagining it. It's easy to get defensive over such claims, we've all been there! But I think once we understand the mechanism of pain and the brain, it's easier to explain to people however frustrating it may seem that our pain is real.

This does lead me to to ask you to take an honest look at how you are emotionally right now or were at the start of your pain journey? Did it begin at a time when you were experiencing higher stress levels? After a trauma? Or do you suffer with depression or anxiety? By all means this book will still help and give you practical help with your pain, but you will see greater improvement by addressing the mental health issue underlying the cause of your pain.

Pain signals are caused by a release of chemicals called neurotransmitters. Scientists have identified over a hundred different neurotransmitters. Some of them reduce pain (good neurotransmitters the most common being endorphins), and some of them increase pain (bad neurotransmitters, the most common being cortisol). Again the release of these neurotransmitters is often controlled by our emotions. Things which we enjoy result in the release of good neurotransmitters such as laughing with a friend, eating our favourite foods or having a treatment such as massage or reflexology. Whilst things which we do not enjoy or being angry or irritable can release bad neurotransmitters. Being in pain itself can cause the release of more bad neurotransmitters and so the cycle continues. Pain medication usually works by promoting good neurotransmitters or blocking the release of bad neurotransmitters. This is why doctors often prescribe anti-depressants for chronic conditions. I know there is often a reluctance to take such medications; partly because it feeds into the 'it's all in your head' stigma. But like all approaches, if they give you the kick-start you need to start your recovery, then surely they are worth a try.

Hopefully you now have a better understanding of pain, what causes it and the chemistry involved in increasing or decreasing it. Armed with this knowledge the mind-pain association becomes easy to recognise and less offensive. It also may help you in formulating ideas to reduce your bad neurotransmitters and increase your good neurotransmitters.

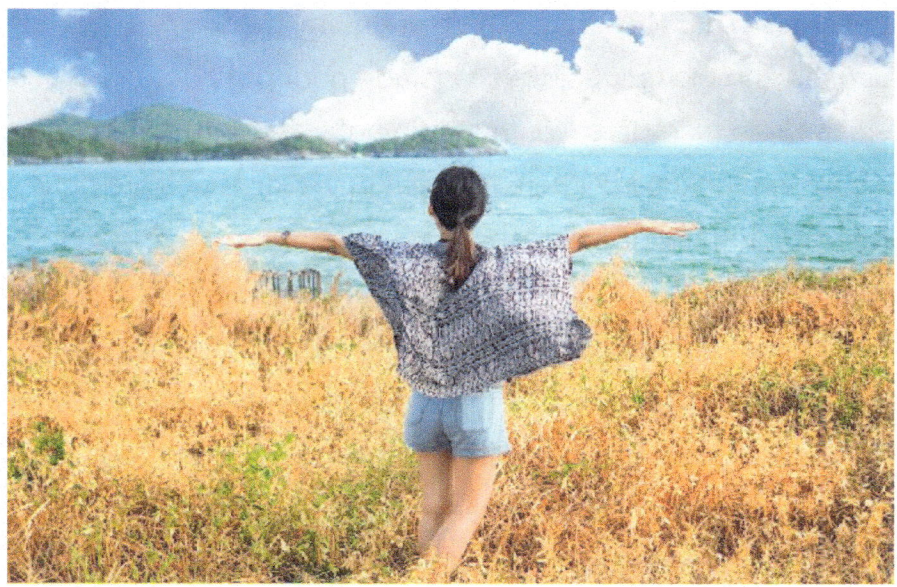

© Dark caramel dreamstime.com

Moving onto chronic fatigue, characterised as an extreme fatigue, which does not improve with rest or sleep and impacts your daily life. The fatigue is usually worsened and delayed after a period of activity i.e. you feel fatigued the day after an increase in activity rather than straight away. For fatigue to be classified as chronic, it needs to have continued for three months or more.

Treatment is often more complicated as there are many reasons for fatigue and without knowing the real cause (as is usually the case for the conditions we are covering here) it becomes difficult to treat. There are many theories as to what causes chronic fatigue, these include poor gut bacteria, sleep/brain disorders (i.e. the brain not 'resetting' itself during sleep) and unknown viruses. As yet however, these are only theories and nothing has been proven.

For some of you, the cause of your fatigue may be obvious (long Covid for example). However if your fatigue has no known cause it is worth trying to investigate its' origins. Going for endless tests with seemingly no answers may be frustrating, but sometimes ruling out possibilities e.g. nutritional deficiencies is just as important in order to form a treatment plan. Most frustratingly though is that the majority of fatigue has no known cause and therefore treating it becomes trial and error and down to the individual. This book contains the most widely accepted methods to improve fatigue, but as with pain, there is no miracle cure and what works for one person may not work for another.

We are probably all guilty of dismissing our fatigue to others as 'tiredness'. We probably do so because we don't want to be seen as complaining or hoping the other person can relate. To do so however is an injustice. True fatigue cannot compare to simply being tired and actually leaves people thinking we just need a good night's sleep; if only it were that simple!

Not only does true fatigue become physically debilitating but it becomes mentally tiring too. Often cited as 'brain fog' it becomes difficult to think or concentrate clearly. You may also become forgetful and confused.

If you take one piece of advice from this book it is to start differentiating between being tired and being fatigued. Ensuring you get a good night's sleep is one of the top recommendations for improving fatigue and so recognising the difference for yourself means you will know if this is an issue for you. Being clear with other people, means they can understand and support you better. You may think you are sparing their feelings, but you need to be surrounded by people who understand your condition and will love and care for you during your bad days too, that can only happen if you are honest.

It's easy to see from this introduction how difficult it is to treat pain and fatigue related conditions. With scientists unclear on what causes such conditions and very little research, how can we expect to be cured? What is clear, is that these conditions vary between individuals, meaning a personalised approach to treatment is needed, something the majority of the medical community simply don't have the time or resources to offer. I hope in the following pages, you will find some advice and resources to better manage your own condition. Not all of the methods may help you, that is ok, simply move onto something else. But learning your body and what does benefit you, will hopefully set you on a healthier, energetic and pain free path.

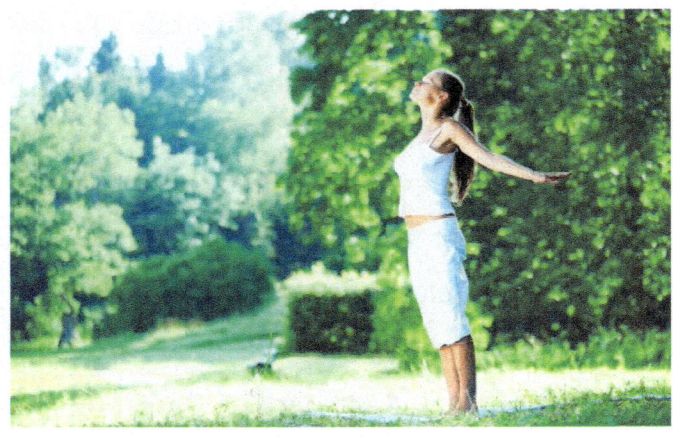

©Ivan Mikhaylov dreamstime.com

Know Your Triggers

One of the most frustrating aspects of living with a pain or fatigue disorder is the uncertainty. One day you may appear 'well' and able to live a 'normal' life, whilst the next you need to take to your bed.

For some people the reason for their flare-ups or bad days may be obvious. Those who have lived with a condition for a while may have discovered their triggers. For some, especially those newly diagnosed it can be difficult to identify their triggers as so many variables are possible. Diet and stress are two of the main possibilities and arguably the easiest culprits to control ourselves. However, some triggers are beyond our control, for example I have clients (particularly Arthritis and Fibromyalgia clients) tell me damp, cold weather affects them.

Of course not much can be done about the weather (other than maybe taking a holiday in the winter rather than the summer months!). But if you know your triggers, they become easier to avoid or you can put a plan in place to manage them and hopefully prevent flare-ups.

Some other possible triggers to be aware of include;

- Lack of sleep
- Lack of exercise
- Dehydration
- Medications
- Being overweight
- Too much alcohol, caffeine or drugs.

This list is not exhaustive and will vary for each person. If you need help identifying your triggers, I've included a tracker in the worksheet section. You will probably need to continue the tracker for longer than a week, maybe even a few months to get a clear idea so feel free to photocopy/print out several copies and keep in a folder.

Exercise

I know what you're thinking! When you are in pain or fatigued to the point you can barely move, exercise is the last thing on your mind! However, hear me out. No-one is expecting you to do a full gym workout or compete in a marathon. Exercise in this instance can be any movement which increases your activity. If that means walking around the garden twice instead of once, then that counts!

We all know that the benefits of exercise are plentiful. From increasing circulation and therefore strengthening the heart, keeping strong and supple in later life and the mental health benefits. However when starting from being sedentary, it is important to gradually increase activity. Pushing yourself too much often results in set backs and an increase in symptoms the next day.

I try not to get too weighed down with science in these guides however, I do think it is important that we understand the role of the lymphatic system in relation to fatigue. Simply speaking, the lymphatic system is the network in our body which moves lymph throughout. Lymph is the fluid which transports nutrients to cells and takes back waste material to be excreted. It is also heavily associated with our immune system, transporting immune cells which fight infections. Unlike the circulation system, the lymphatic system doesn't have an organ like the heart to pump this fluid around our body. Instead it relies largely on our own movement and muscle contraction to move this fluid. If symptoms have made us become largely sedentary, the flow of lymph becomes slower. Without sufficient lymphatic flow, lymph can become stagnant, causing poor immune response, puffy areas (especially ankles), and feeling sluggish, thereby continuing the fatigue cycle. It is easy to conclude therefore that any movement can contribute to moving lymph, thus helping the body to work more efficiently. So next time you're struggling with the simplest of activity, try to see the bigger picture and just a small push of, for example moving to a different room, taking some stretches, rotating your ankles and wrists, all help to increase lymph flow, which in turn should help you feel better and allow you to do more the next day. Other activities you could try to improve lymphatic flow include Lymphatic Drainage Massage; a specialist massage technique to specifically target the Lymphatic System (although I would argue any massage would aid the Lymphatic System if you struggle to find someone trained in your area), and dry body brushing; using a bristle brush, apply long sweeping strokes, towards the heart i.e. start at the wrists/ankles towards the shoulder/groin.

Rather than recommending exercise for both pain and fatigue, I propose we focus instead on the term movement. Movement, however small can still be advantageous, and mentally is much more achievable. Simple stretching and low-impact, light movement prevents joints and muscles from seizing and stiffening up, which can continue the cycle of pain, especially in conditions like Arthritis.

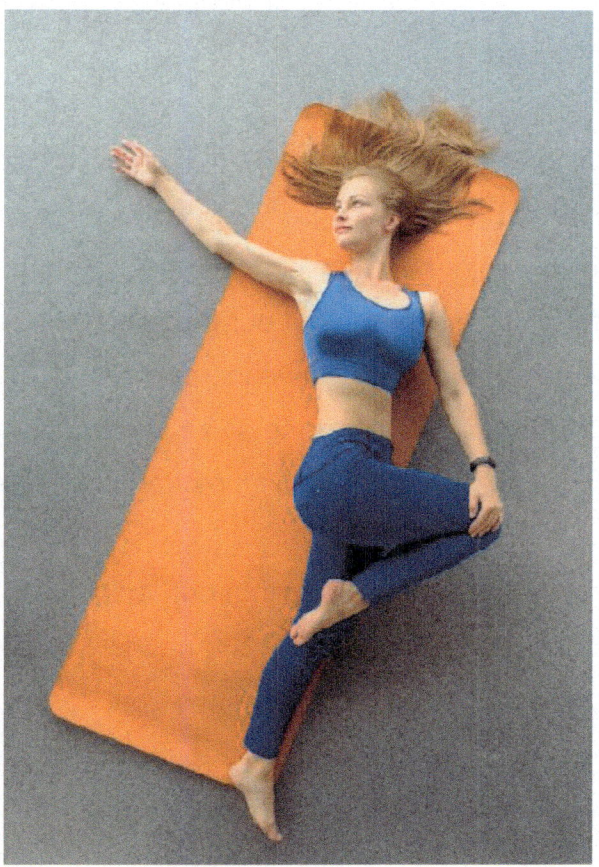

© Denys Kurbatov Dreamstime.com

www.leru-wellness.co.uk

The term functional movement is often used when describing a rehabilitation plan. Functional movement looks at everyday tasks which you find difficult, and aims to improve your ability to complete them. Start by analysing tasks you find difficult and would like to improve e.g. bending down to put your shoes on, opening a jar, washing or brushing your hair. Score the task on whether you can complete it and how painful it is. This now becomes your benchmark so you can assess any improvement.

I understand the temptation that when a task causes you pain, you avoid doing it. I agree in principle, I'm not a fan of the no-pain-no-gain mentality either. Inflicting pain on an already painful muscle only makes our muscles tense up further, causing us more pain. However, avoiding doing something can also only serve us to seize up and increase pain further, after all we can't avoid all movement in life.

Instead, we need to work within our limits and gradually increase our repetition. Let's take the example of struggling to bend down and put our shoes on. A simple easy exercise to help improve that would be to bend down and touch our toes. Maybe when you first try, you can only reach down as far as your knees. That's fine, repeat that movement until you start to feel fatigued, maybe that's ten repetitions. Now we have a base level. The next day, either try to stretch a little further or increase the number of repetitions, even if only by one. Always keep within your comfort level and stop if you get any pain. Keep repeating this exercise daily and within time you will hopefully see an improvement in your chosen activity.

Once you see improvements in your functional movement, it is then time to move on to more generic exercises. Again, I'm not talking about heavy intensive workouts, start small with low-impact stretches. You don't even need to go to a class, there are plenty of yoga and pilates videos on Youtube, many of which are relatively short at less than fifteen minutes. Another benefit of home workouts, is that you can take them at your own pace, pause or stop at anytime with no judgement and no panicking how you're going to get home after using up all of your energy.

The usual guidance on exercise for chronic pain and fatigue is often low-impact exercises such as yoga and pilates. Whilst these can be effective for some, for some of us with chronic conditions they can be too intense, particularly if you are completely new to these kind of exercises and lack the flexibility and core-strength needed. Personally, I have found Tai Chi to be much more beneficial for our circumstances and largely under-rated. Tai Chi originates from China and involves slow, repetitive, almost meditative movements. It puts less pressure on the joints than yoga and stretches, instead helping to keep joints supple. It is ideal for beginners as is suitable for all fitness levels. I've also found it to be beneficial for improving balance, co-ordination and brain-fog/concentration, so is a great one to try if you struggle with fatigue. Again if there are no classes near you or you find that prospect too daunting, then there are plenty of instructional videos on Youtube.

Living with a chronic condition often means we stay at home too much and become quite isolated which can wreak havoc with our mental health. Exercising outdoors if you can, can be particularly advantageous. Ideally being around nature such as a walk in a park or by a river, helps to promote those good neurotransmitters and is so beneficial for our mental health. If you live in a city, just walking round the block can still help. Take the time to absorb the sights, sounds and smells of being outdoors.

Whatever activity you choose, the most important thing is for it to be a form of exercise you enjoy. If exercise feels like a chore it is not going to boost those neurotransmitters and only promote anxiety, procrastination and feelings of being incapable. We are therefore much less likely to continue with it.

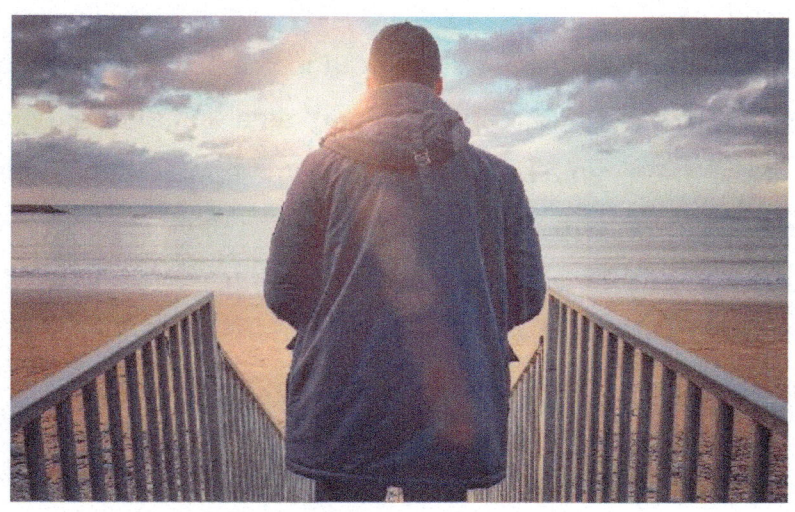

© Creativecommonsstockphotos dreamstime.com

Previously, graduated exercise plans were recommended for people with Chronic Fatigue, however this has been largely discredited in recent years. Personally I believe, as previously stated no one thing can 'cure' you. Too much emphasis was placed on these programs without taking a holistic approach. I do believe graduated exercise has its' place, so long as the program is not too regimented. If you are having a bad day, exercising through it is not going to benefit; if you need to rest, rest. You can always go back to your regime once you are feeling better.

In chronic fatigue circles you may also hear the phrase 'Spoon Theory' being passed around. The term was first coined by writer Christine Miserandino in 2003 and is designed to give a visual representation of how much energy a person has. If we imagine a 'spoon' as a unit of energy, then tasks can be given a rating of how many 'spoons' they would use. On a low energy day, a person would have less spoons to spend and therefore manage and prioritise their activity. Whilst I can see the benefits for some people i.e. the organised type of person, for me it over complicates

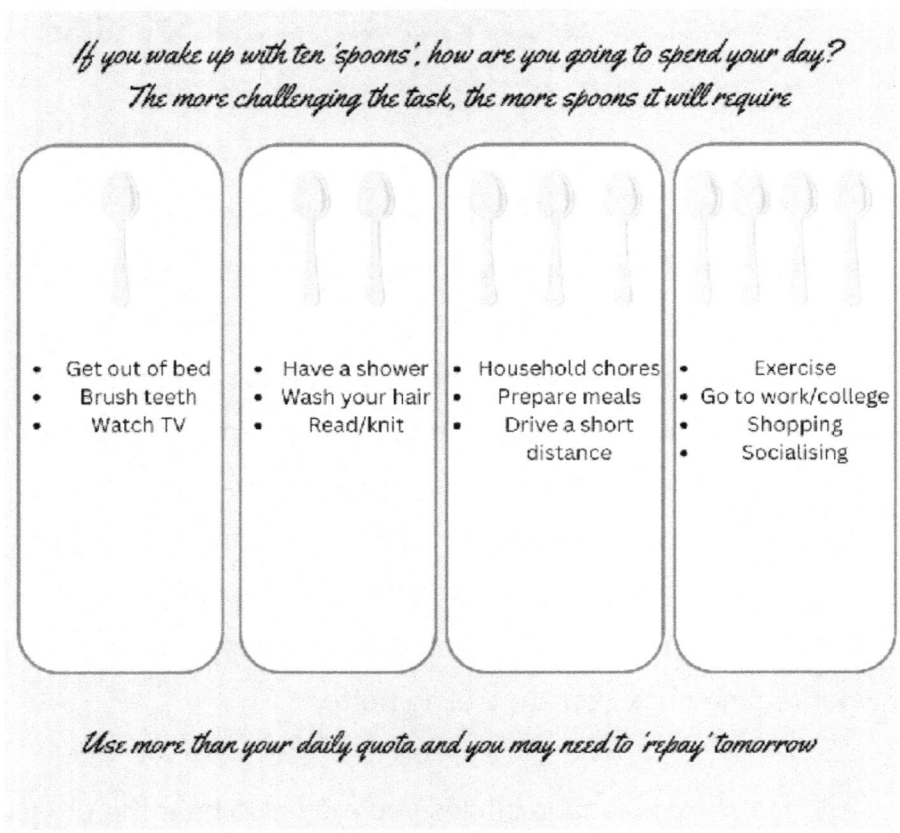

A guide to Spoon theory and assigning activity to spoon amounts

something which should come naturally. Where I do think it has benefit, is in explaining our fatigue and how it can vary daily to our loved ones or other non-sufferers. If a partner or kids for example, know it's a 'three-spoon day' then they can make allowances and not put you under pressure for not being at your best.

When you have a condition which changes daily (and often within each day), sticking to a strict plan just isn't achievable for many. Instead, keeping a track of daily activity is likely more beneficial. That way you can track your progress, and have a clear idea of when and by how much to increase activity. Include how an activity made you feel, if it repeatedly exacerbates your symptoms it may be that you need to drop it from your routine.

Beginning any exercise routine is often the most difficult part, even for healthy people. It is easy to make excuses when we don't see instant results. Exercise can feel like a commitment and take motivation we simply don't have. However, time for some tough love again; if you want to see changes, only you can put in the effort. It takes on average 66 days to form a new habit, although this figure can vary between 18 and 254 [1]. Therefore when starting a routine, it is important to try and stick with it as much as you can. Once exercise forms your routine, you should find that you will miss it if you stop.

Looking after your Mental Health

Thankfully in recent years the stigma associated with mental health is subsiding. However, some people particularly the older ones amongst us still feel embarrassed or ashamed to admit we are struggling. Mental health issues do not discriminate and can afflict anyone, but for those living with a chronic condition they are even more prevalent. It is even more important therefore, to look after our mental health, and as we've already discussed promoting these good neurotransmitters, could have a knock-on affect of improving our symptoms.

The over-riding conclusion of coping mentally with a chronic condition is that of acceptance. There are many things in life which we cannot control, and those of us with chronic conditions understand this all too well. Learning to accept that which we cannot control i.e. our condition, can take time and be frustrating. I'm a strong believer in looking for positives in situations; what is the lesson I can take from my condition? How is this going to make me a stronger person? Perhaps it will make you a more empathetic or resilient individual. Or will it make you re-evaluate your career or relationships for the better?

www.leru-wellness.co.uk

Practising daily gratitude is a good way to focus on the positives of your situation and learn acceptance. If you journal or keep a diary, start making a point of including one thing which happened each day which you are grateful for. It can be as simple as getting dressed or leaving the house. Hopefully as you progress your gratitude will be less about your condition and more about your life, loved ones and things you enjoy. If you don't keep a journal, try writing your daily gratitude on a piece of paper and store in a jar or small box to look over at a later date (on a bad day for example). Once you get into the habit of observing gratitude daily, it becomes one piece in the puzzle of achieving a more positive outlook.

Recently there has been talk on Social Media of looking for 'glimmers' to help with mental health. Similar to recognising gratitude in increasing positivity; glimmers are small things which we enjoy that makes us appreciate and see the beauty in our life. Examples can include a sunset, listening to bird song, favourite foods, a song which holds a dear memory. Look out for glimmers in your daily life and add them to your daily gratitude.

Daily affirmations are another popular way to increase positivity in our lives. Based on the principle; what we believe we become, adding a positive thought or wish into our daily rituals is another form of positive goal setting and helps to accept our situation. If you struggle with the idea of affirmations, try to think of them in the opposite way. That is, when we dwell on negativity, more negativity arises. Have you ever noticed how bad situations all seem to happen at once, almost like the world is conspiring against you? From minor annoyances such as already running late and being met with a traffic jam which makes us even later? Right through to more serious situations like ill health or grief. In reality, when we are stressed we become increasingly aware of more stressors which causes us to spiral into negativity. If we reverse this, we can conclude that acknowledging positivity and gratitude, only promotes more positivity.

Getting into the mindset of affirmations can take practice. I've included some examples on the following pages. Use them however is right for you; recite them in your head or out loud, photocopy them and add them to your journal, laminate them and post them on your fridge or your office. Whichever serves as a daily reminder for you. Feel free to add your own but remember to avoid any negative language.

www.leru-wellness.co.uk

affirmation CARDS

Print these affirmation cards to help you shift your mindset and achieve your dream goals. Begin your day with positive intentions. You can laminate the cards or print them on cardstock, hang the affirmation cards on your wall or add them to your planner.

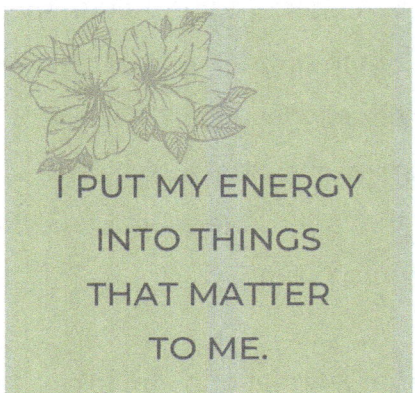

I PUT MY ENERGY INTO THINGS THAT MATTER TO ME.

I GIVE MYSELF PERMISSION TO DO WHAT IS RIGHT FOR ME.

I AM BECOMING CLOSER TO MY TRUE SELF EVERY DAY.

I AM AT PEACE WITH WHO I AM AS A PERSON.

affirmation CARDS

Print these affirmation cards to help you shift your mindset and achieve your dream goals. Begin your day with positive intentions.
You can laminate the cards or print them on cardstock, hang the affirmation cards on your wall or add them to your planner.

EVERY DAY I AM GETTING HEALTHIER AND STRONGER.

BEING HAPPY COMES EASY TO ME. HAPPINESS IS MY SECOND NATURE.

GOOD THINGS ARE HAPPENING.

I AM DEEPLY FULFILLED BY WHAT I DO.

www.leru-wellness.co.uk

affirmation CARDS

Print these affirmation cards to help you shift your mindset and achieve your dream goals. Begin your day with positive intentions. You can laminate the cards or print them on cardstock, hang the affirmation cards on your wall or add them to your planner.

I DESERVE TO BE HEALTHY AND FEEL GOOD.

I AM IN THE PROCESS OF BECOMING THE BEST VERSION OF MYSELF.

MY POSSIBILITIES ARE ENDLESS.

I BELIEVE I CAN BE ALL THAT I WANT TO BE.

The unpredictable nature of living with a chronic condition means there will be days which are more difficult than others. Developing a plan and prioritising tasks should help with the overwhelm. As with exercise, if you are having a bad day and really not up to doing much then go with it! If your body needs an afternoon of laying on the sofa and doing very little, then don't fight it. Carrying on when you are truly burnt out will only cause a setback later. Be kinder to yourself and normalise rest days, they are an important part of recovery. If that means you need to include one or more a week into your diary then so be it. If that's really not possible, break down tasks into smaller, more manageable chunks of time, with plenty of breaks in-between. Alternatively, delegate tasks to others.

Once stress and anxiety take hold, left untreated they can very quickly spiral into depression. The more self-care you can add into your daily routine, the less likely that will happen as it gives the mind something else to focus. Having a purpose in life, goals and ambition is paramount to preventing a downwards spiral in mental health.

Goal setting can be split into two parts; long-term and short term. Both are usually of equal importance. Setting long-term plans such as career, family, travelling may take much more consideration when living with a chronic

www.leru-wellness.co.uk

condition. But it is vital that you have focus, something achievable for you in order to drive you to improve your health.

Similar to glimmers, short-term goals add value and joy to our day to day life. In this instance, they will probably be focused around hobbies, volunteering or connecting with friends and family.

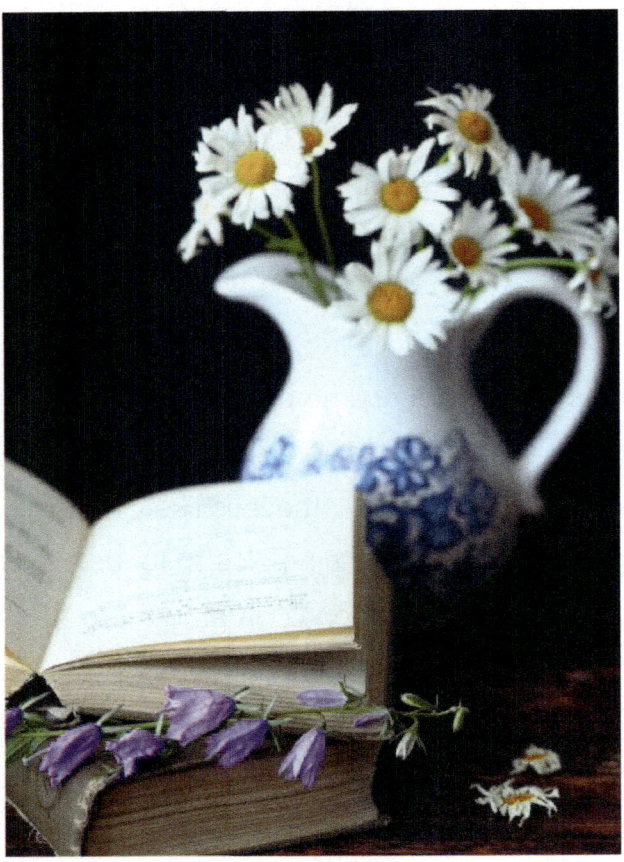

© Jolijuli Dreamstime.com

Not only can hobbies provide stress-relief, they can act as a distraction to any physical symptoms. Have you ever noticed how your pain feels worse when in bed at night or crashed out on the sofa? Yet if you have a full and busy day they've not been so bad? Hobbies can also have the same impact. Obviously consideration needs to be given to the physicality, but there are things you can enjoy which do not involve too much physical exertion. Examples include;

- Arts and crafts
- Reading
- Learning a musical instrument
- Learning a new language

Often when we struggle with our mental health, we become very insular, too focused on ourselves. Volunteering is a great way to step back and give your attention to someone else. Again, it doesn't have to be physical, many charities now for example have opportunities on the phone whereby you call someone and are a listening ear for them. I don't really like the cliche of 'there is always someone worse off than you' but it is humbling to realise that others have different challenges and there is a great sense of satisfaction knowing you have made someone else's day a little brighter.

Looking after your mental health, like a lot of the advice in this book, isn't something that can be done once, or occasionally. It requires a commitment of daily practice in order to create a new habit or new way of thinking. In addition to those already listed, incorporating one or more of the following (free!) self-care rituals into your daily routine should improve your overall well-being by boosting those good neurotransmitters;

- Meditation or other breathing techniques
- Baths
- Giving yourself a mini-facial
- Painting your nails
- Call a friend you haven't spoken to in a while
- Create a playlist of your favourite/uplifting songs
- Watch your favourite movie

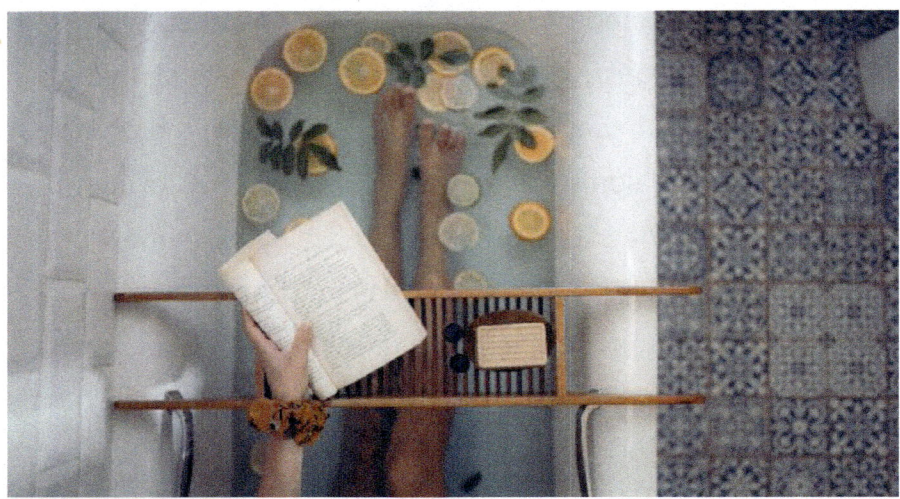

Again, this is about boosting those neurotransmitters, so like exercise, in order to be beneficial needs to be something you enjoy.

If self-help stress management techniques aren't working for you and you are still struggling, I do urge you to seek the help of a qualified counsellor. Talking to friends and family is of course beneficial, but sometimes talking to a neutral person without judgement, who we don't know, allows us to be more honest. Plus the guidance you will gain from an experienced professional should be unsurpassed.

You may also gain comfort from seeking out support groups (both in person and online) from others who suffer from the same conditions. No-one understands what you are going through more than a fellow sufferer. A basic internet search will bring up the many national charities and Facebook groups covering every condition, or your health care provider may be able to point you in the direction of local centres or charities. However alone you may feel, there is help out there, sometimes you just need to be pro-active in your search for it.

Cryo- and Heat Therapy

Cryotherapy simply means applying cold as a form of treatment. Putting ice on an injury is nothing new, however, thanks to Wim Hof, Cryotherapy in the form of ice baths has become fashionable of late. I know these aren't for everyone and so I'm going to cover some other ways cryotherapy may be beneficial for you. Some may benefit from applying heat instead and so in this chapter we'll also cover when you could consider this.

There have been numerous studies showing the benefits of Cryotherapy including pain reduction, muscle healing, reduction in inflammation and reduction in anxiety and depression. Research in this area however is new and further studies are needed. From my reading and experience, it does seem promising for improving many pain/fatigue related issues and is certainly worth experimenting to see if it benefits you.

If you are wanting to give ice baths a try, I do recommend having a look at Wim Hof's website or app. There are lots of exercises to get you started and gradually get used to colder temperatures, please do not be tempted to plunge straight into icy waters with no preparation!. His website also

www.leru-wellness.co.uk

contains lots of research on the benefits of ice baths, including improving various pain and fatigue conditions. Just read with an open mind and remember we all respond differently, just because ice baths are one person's miracle cure, unfortunately they are not everyone's.

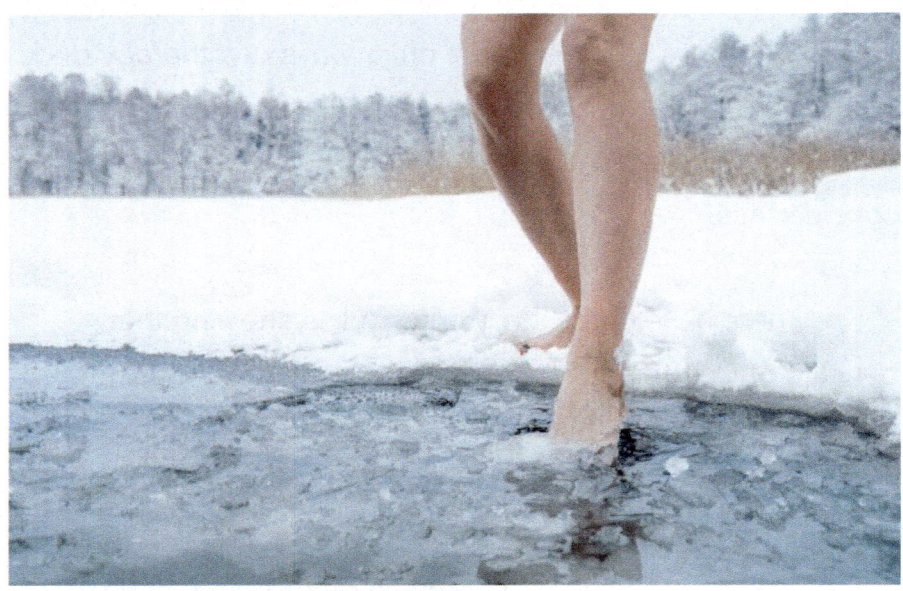

If you're not feeling brave enough to try or have the money to buy an ice bath, then consider turning your shower to cold for the final ten seconds or so. In fact this is advised as a starting exercise for ice baths. Yes, it may feel intolerable but take some deep breaths and after a short while your body will get used to the temperature. Afterwards, notice how you feel. How are your energy levels? Do you have any pain? Is there a reduction in pain? Personally, I've found after a shower I often need to sit down for ten minutes or so as the heat wipes me out. Turning the heat down gives me a rush of endorphins, meaning I have more energy and no longer need to rest. It has now become part of my routine, so although I dread turning the temperature dial down, I'd miss it if I stopped!

Some spas and clinics have Cryo ice chambers. These are similar to ice baths, a person would sit in them for a couple of minutes and allow the body to cool to a lower temperature. They are ideal if you feel nervous about giving Cryotherapy a try as you will have a trained person to assist you and also give you a chance to try before buying an ice bath. However, ideally you should be using these chambers regularly to reap the most benefit which could prove costy.

There are also targeted Cryotherapy machines whereby a practitioner will apply a cold stream to a single area of the body. These are ideal for an injury, inflammation or isolated painful areas, arthritis for example. Usually a course of treatments will be recommended and in chronic conditions such as arthritis regular maintenance sessions may be advised. Again this could prove costly for some but are ideal if you want the benefits of cryotherapy but don't want the full body exposure.

Cold therapy, whether an at home DIY ice bath, cold water swimming or a professional led treatment is not recommended if you are pregnant or have a heart condition. If you have any other health concerns you may wish to consult with your health care provider before trying cryotherapy.

For some pain issues, applying heat can be beneficial. Applying a hot water bottle or heat pad to an area of tight, stiff muscles or if in spasm can help to loosen them up. Heat is usually recommended for long-term pain issues, 48 hours after an injury and if no inflammation is present. Sometimes heat can exacerbate conditions like arthritis (due to the inflammation) so proceed with caution.

Generally, I would not recommend too much heat for those of us with fatigue related conditions, in fact chronic fatigue is a contra-indication for hot stone massage as it can exacerbate the condition. For that reason I would also recommend caution when using saunas and steam rooms too, particularly if you are having a flare-up or a bad day. Isolated heat such as a hot water bottle should be fine, just be careful of too much heat to the full body. If you do wish to partake in hot tubs, saunas etc, keep sessions shorter.

Nutrition

I am by no means a nutritionist, however I do feel it important to include a chapter on nutrition in this book. What we eat is so important for our energy levels and can have a huge significance on our physical health, it would be remiss of me to overlook nutrition as a way to improve any pain and fatigue condition.

When it comes to nutrition especially, I believe in a personalised approach. We all have different needs based on our activity levels, medication, gut microbiome and even our personal tastes and intolerances that getting the right nutrition to deal with a chronic condition becomes too complex for your generic online or influencer advice. So if you are looking to get serious and make drastic changes to your diet, then I encourage you to seek out a consultation with a fully qualified and accredited nutritionist. Unfortunately due to the rising popularity of social media influencers and no accreditation of nutritionists, there are people out there claiming to be nutritionists with little more than a weekend course which only covered weight loss. Make sure therefore that the person you choose is trained to at least degree level and is ideally on your nations register if applicable (for the UK this would be BANT).

With that in mind, the following advice is largely from my own experience and research, it is not meant to be exhaustive or overly complicated. If you take one piece of advice from this chapter, it is to eat a balanced diet containing lots of fruits and vegetables with as little processed foods as possible, which if we're being honest is advice we all should be following and have probably heard a million times before!

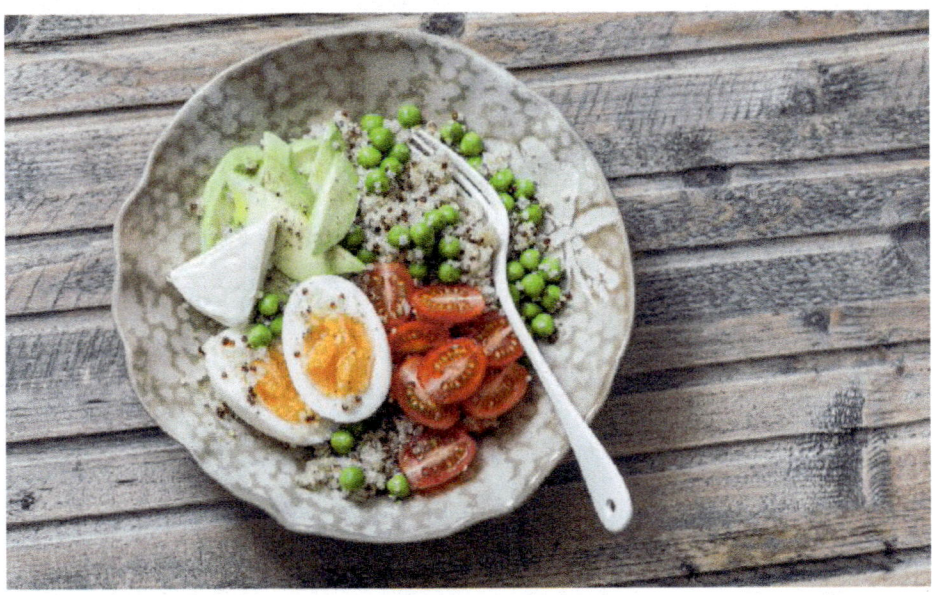

© Oksana Kiian Dreamstime.com

Whilst I'm not trying to body-shame here, I fully embrace the body positive movement and acceptance of all shapes and sizes, from a health perspective being overweight will not help your situation. Carrying excess pounds puts extra strain on the joints, making them more painful. It also means the body becomes fatigued more easily since carrying round extra weight requires more energy. So if you are overweight, then trying to lose some will benefit your condition. Following a balanced diet rather than a miracle quick-fix, is the best and safest way for long-term, sustainable weight loss.

Around 10% of our calorie intake is used by the digestive system to break down said food into energy. Some foods such as protein can use even more, up to 30%. If we are struggling with fatigue, it makes sense therefore in order to conserve energy, to eat foods which are easier to digest. This is possibly one of the reasons why Irritable Bowel symptoms are often present in conditions like Fibromyalgia and Chronic Fatigue. Our bodies simply don't have the energy needed for digestion, or are preserving the little energy we do have and so food isn't broken down properly resulting in symptoms such as bloating, constipation and diarrhoea. This digestive process is often the reason we may get an energy slump after a large meal. If so, you may benefit from switching

www.leru-wellness.co.uk

from eating three large meals a day to more (5-6), smaller meals evenly spaced, or even grazing throughout the day.

If your condition is giving irritable bowel symptoms also then it is generally advised to cut down on fried, fatty foods, spicy foods, alcohol and fizzy drinks particularly those containing artificial sweeteners. These items are difficult to digest, give us little in terms of nutrition and vitamins, and can lead to gastro issues. Personally I'd also add foods with added protein (protein bars, powders etc) to that list. As we've already seen, protein takes a lot of energy to break down and a lot of these supplements irritate the digestive system. Instead, I'd suggest getting your protein intake from unprocessed and so easier to digest sources, such as lean meats, nuts, tofu, eggs and dairy. I'm not suggesting protein is 'bad'. We do need some for muscle repair, growth and it actually helps us to keep full for longer so can help with weight management as we eat less total calories. But, unless you are an athlete or trying to gain muscle mass, these added protein, processed foods serve little purpose and could actually be hindering your digestion and energy resources.

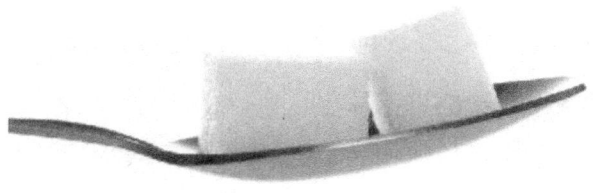

© Chris Brignall Dreamstime.com

Sugar has received bad press in recent years and on researching, it is easy to see why. Food-wise it is the biggest zapper of energy, creating a sugar-high which then comes crashing down causing our energy levels to crash. And our bodies response? Crave more of the sweet stuff, causing the cycle to continue. Unfortunately sugar is addictive, meaning you can try and cut down, but to really break the cycle a full sugar detox will give you the best results.

Sugar is not only the villain in causing havoc with our energy, it is also believed to increase inflammation in the body [2], thus leading to pain and conditions such as arthritis. If you are going to look into changing your diet to improve symptoms, I cannot stress enough how looking at your sugar intake should be your first priority. Unfortunately, whilst you may not think you have a sweet tooth or drink soft drinks,

www.leru-wellness.co.uk

sugar is hidden in most processed foods including; pasta and curry sauces, ketchup, soups and baked beans. If you are serious about breaking your sugar habit, I highly recommend you look up Sarah Wilson's 'I Quit Sugar' program and website, this is the plan I used to break my own sugar addiction. It is not a 'fad' diet, rather a plan for clean, unprocessed eating, and unlike many sugar nay-sayers, still allows you to eat carbs!

None of us are perfect when it comes to our diets and I'm not a fan of being too regimented with what we eat. Eating completely unprocessed, zero-sugar, low trans-fats is unsustainable and quite frankly boring in today's lifestyle. Aiming to eat healthily for the majority of the time and not denying ourselves an occasional treat is key to keeping momentum with any healthy eating plan. Instead of feeling guilty over any misdemeanour, use it as a learning experience. How did eating that chocolate brownie really make me feel? Did I notice an energy slump? How has it sat in my stomach? Am I noticing an increase in pain symptoms afterwards? And most importantly; was it worth the symptoms I'm now feeling? By following these questions you will gain a clearer insight into how foods affect your symptoms so that next time you're tempted, if it's a food you know makes you feel dreadful, you will be more likely to say no or at least be prepared for any consequences!

We all know that we should be eating more fruits and vegetables. Current UK guidelines state that we should consume at least thirty different plant-based foods each week, so four to five a day on average. The key here is *different* fruits and vegetables. If we eat the same foods everyday we are not getting enough of a variety of different vitamins and minerals. By all means eat an apple a day if you wish, but it will only count as one towards your weekly goal of thirty. These guidelines are updated from the previous 'five a day' which only covered fruits and vegetables. The new thirty plant foods is actually more flexible as it includes grains such as oats and quinoa, nuts and seeds and even chocolate! (Providing it is minimum 70% cocoa).

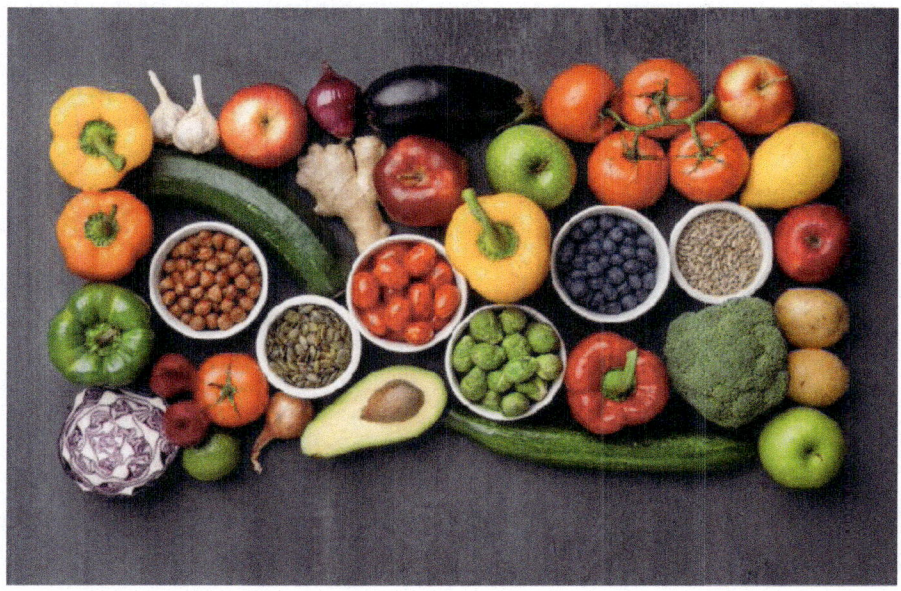

© Shmeljov **dreamstime.com**

Many people benefit from incorporating juices or smoothies into their diet. The process breaks down the fibre making the fruits and vegetables easier to digest. This does mean they cannot be included in our 'thirty varieties a week' quota. However, many would argue that it is still a good way to get lots of vitamins as they usually contain several fruits and vegetables. Also breaking down the fibre can actually make them easier to digest for many so maybe worth replacing breakfast for example with a smoothie for a week and see if it benefits you. Just be careful of recipes which contain only fruit. You wouldn't eat for example, half a pineapple, three bananas, a mango and six oranges in one sitting, the sugar hit would be intense! Yet because the drink only contains fruit and natural ingredients people still think this is healthy. Sugar is sugar, despite it coming from a natural source. Try to lean more towards smoothies which have some veggies in or the sugar comes from mainly apples and berries rather than high sugar fruits.

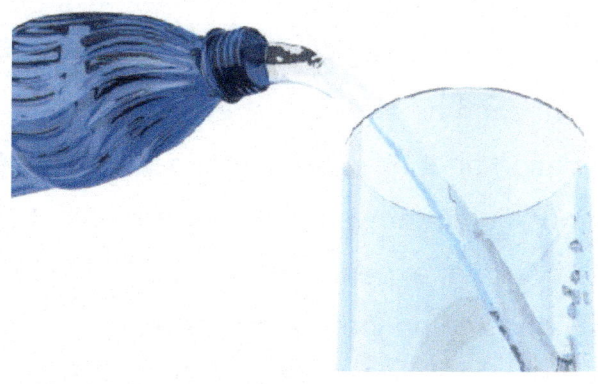

© Alexsandr Golovashchenko Dreamstime.com

Keeping hydrated with plenty of water is another activity we all know we should be doing, but very few of us actually do. It doesn't help with no clear advice or evidence as to how much we should all be drinking. We do know however that dehydration can cause symptoms associated with pain and fatigue. In terms of pain, drinking water helps to lubricate our joints which act as shock-absorbers. Without this lubrication, joint pain becomes an issue. We also know that dehydration can affect brain function which can lead to a reduction in cognitive skills and memory (I.e. brain fog). If increasing water intake can also improve athletic performance [3], it stands to reason that improving hydration should also help chronic fatigue too.

The majority of us aim, or at least have been conditioned to believe, we should be drinking around eight glasses of water a day. However there is controversy around that claim with no real evidence to show it is accurate. As with all things health, each person will have their own optimum amount based on their size, activity and climate (I.e. we need to drink more in hotter weather). Pay attention to how much you are drinking, experiment by increasing intake by a glass or two a day and notice if it improves your symptoms, particularly headaches and muscle cramps; two of the most common signs of dehydration. You can then use this experiment to create your own optimum daily intake.

As I've said before, I'm not a believer in sticking to strict diet plans. Variety and keeping indulgent foods to occasion is key to maintaining a healthy eating plan long-term. However there are certain foods which have been shown to reduce inflammation (and therefore pain) and improve energy levels. By adding these items into your daily intake, you may find an improvement.

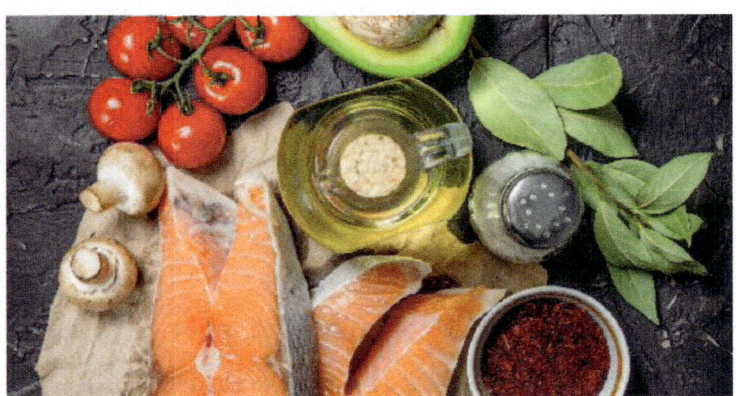

©Olesya1041sh dreamstime.com

Top five foods for Reducing Inflammation

1/ Omega-3 rich foods including oily fish such as salmon or mackerel and flax seed.

2/ Berries such as blueberries, strawberries and cherries. These contain a high level of antioxidants to counteract inflammation. Cherries, particularly cherry juice has been shown to help with inflammation and muscle pain [4]

3/ Nuts and seeds, especially walnuts and almonds which have a good amount of healthy fats.

4/ Turmeric. If you're not a fan of curries this spice is also commonly available as a supplement which many swear by for helping with arthritis pain

5/ Ginger. Studies have shown ginger to be good for reducing inflammation and also for reducing pain, possibly because it helps to improve circulation. It is also readily available as a tea if you struggle to incorporate it into your diet.

Top five foods for Fighting Fatigue

In terms of fighting fatigue, we've already mentioned that sugar is probably the biggest no-no. Instead it needs to be replaced with complex carbohydrates (think wholegrain breads, pastas, rice) and proteins. These keep us full and release energy more slowly meaning they help to stabilise our energy levels. In addition try including the following regularly;

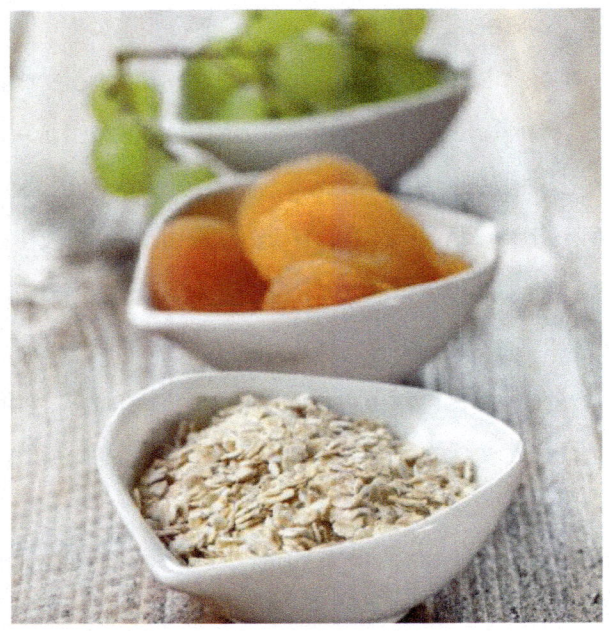

©Corinna Guissemann Dreamstime.com

1/ Oats. A complex carbohydrate which also contains fibre and is anti-inflammatory. Oats will keep you full till lunchtime without the nasty sugar spikes.

2/ Eggs. Containing a good amount of protein to stave off sugar cravings. Eggs are also a good source of Vitamin B12, a deficiency of which can lead to fatigue and brain fog.

3/ Omega-3's from oily fish and walnuts. One for both lists, these healthy fats and proteins release energy slowly and keep us full

4/ Beans. Not only do they release energy slowly but contain fibre and vitamins such as magnesium

5/ Berries. Another item on both lists, since berries have a lower sugar content than other fruits, they are excellent to satisfy sweet cravings without the sugar spike.

Several studies have linked ME to the gut microbiome [5]. Research on this and the gut microbiome in general is still in its infancy and so is too early to give any definitive recommendations. It is however an interesting development and one I think is worth keeping an eye on over the next few years. Not only could it provide treatment options, but there is also the possibility it could result in testing and better diagnosis.

If you are unaware of the gut microbiome; it is the term used for the microbes, bacteria and fungi which exist in the digestive tract. This fauna is essential to our digestion. Scientists have only relatively recently discovered its existence and research is ongoing into its significance in terms of our health. It is believed each of our gut microbiomes are unique and can be affected by our diet, genetics and environments. Using antibiotics is believed to destroy some of these essential bacterias and this is where researchers believe their usage may cause a host of health issues including ME.

An imbalanced gut microbiome may also result in digestive issues, skin complaints such as eczema or acne or weight issues (e.g. unable to gain or lose weight). If you are experiencing these issues also, it may be worth considering your gut microbiome. There are several probiotics available in health food stores or you can try including fermented foods such as kefir (a sour yoghurt drink) or kimchi into your diet everyday. However, these 'off the shelf' products are designed for general use containing many different strains of bacteria. If you are not getting results with these products, it may be they do not contain the bacteria you are deficient in. In order to be sure you are replacing the bacteria you need, you need to know which bacteria you are deficient in. This involves having a stool test which is currently not available on the NHS and therefore only available with private, unregulated companies. If you really feel you need your microbiome testing, research the tests and companies thoroughly as they can be expensive. Weighing up the cost to how much it may benefit you is a decision only you can make.

Complementary Therapies

It's easy to see why complementary therapies prove popular with people who have been told by the medical community that nothing can be done for them. Desperation and frustration makes us seek out help and answers from other sources. Unfortunately this has caused an increase in charlatans making claims of miracle cures and wonder drugs. Of course new research and treatments are coming out all of the time, but personally I'd be wary of anyone making such wild claims without proof. The following are the current treatments I'd recommend you try. They are much more widely available and credible. Results do vary between individuals so whilst none of these treatments will 'cure' you, they may help to ease symptoms and they will certainly cause you no harm. At best they will give you relief for a couple of days. If you can, use that time productively; get a good nights sleep, do some exercises, catch-up with friends and basically kick-start your bodies own healing process. At the very least you will have an enjoyable hour or so and give you something to look forward to thereby increasing those good neurotransmitters we discussed previously.

A small word of caution, with all treatments sometimes people can feel their symptoms worsen during the following

24-48 hours. I've found this particularly to be the case in people who are already unwell and personally I'm more affected by energy based treatments than the tactile ones i.e. massages. Reacting in this way does not mean the treatment has caused you harm, merely a sign that your body is responding and achieving balance. I mention it because when booking an appointment you may want to choose a day when you are free the following day incase you need to take to your bed.

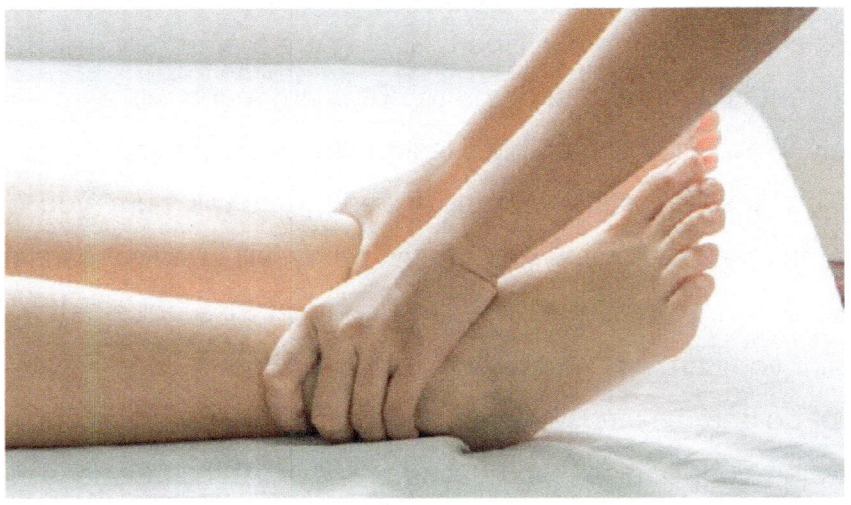

© Srisakorn Wonglakorn Dreamstime.com

Massage

There are over a hundred styles of massage so choosing one which suits can be a minefield. I've mentioned Lymphatic

Drainage before if you are suffering with fatigue and are sedentary. If pain is more your issue it can be tempting to go for a sports/deep tissue/Thai massage however, I've actually found that deeper styles particularly with Fibromyalgia can make pain worse and causes the muscles to tighten further. Less is often more and so I'd actually recommend that you start with a basic Swedish/relaxation massage. Remember the aim for chronic pain is to calm down the nervous system which can be achieved perfectly with relaxation massages. If however, you feel after that you would prefer a deeper style then you can always try that next time. Some useful additions to a Swedish massage may be aromatherapy or hot stones if you can find a practitioner in your area. An aromatherapist will blend some essential oils specifically for you to target your concerns. Communication with your therapist is essential, we are not mind readers so if you feel in pain or that you need them to go deeper then tell them.

Reflexology

Traditionally performed on the feet however versions exist on the hands, face and even ears. This is a pressure point massage in which points on the feet correspond to the rest of the body and so by massaging said points we can affect that part of the body. It can be beneficial for pain relief, as I mentioned above, many in pain cannot bear to be touched in that area so it can help said area without directly touching it. There have been several research papers [6] showing reflexology is effective for pain management and this could be due to it causing the release of the body's own natural painkillers (endorphins i.e. those good neurotransmitters again!).

Learning some simple hand reflexology techniques and reflex locations means you can self-treat as and when needed. The following is an example of a hand reflexology chart. Full disclosure here, incase you are a Reflexology geek and wonder why the reflexes are in different places than where you maybe used to; this is a Korean Hand Therapy chart rather than the hand reflexology charts commonly used in the West and on Google. Having trained in both, and with the Korean version being much more thoroughly researched, it is the version I personally have more faith in.

Hand reflexology is best suited for pain management techniques, but that can also include headaches, period pains and digestive issues. Simply use the chart to match where on the hand you are experiencing pain. The diagram on the following page shows the left hand but you can use the right hand also, it will be a mirror image. If an area is on both hands e.g. a migraine on the left side of your head, then use the left hand, if on the right then use the right hand. Apply pressure on the corresponding part of your hand. This can be in the form of your opposite thumb, using circular massage movements. Or, since the Korean system is based in acupuncture and deeper acupressure techniques, you can be more precise and go deeper using the top of a ball point pen or a knitting needle. Take a couple of deep breaths whilst you maintain the pressure. You may need to move the pressure slightly and experiment a little to get the exact spot, if you've got the right location you should feel relief almost instantly.

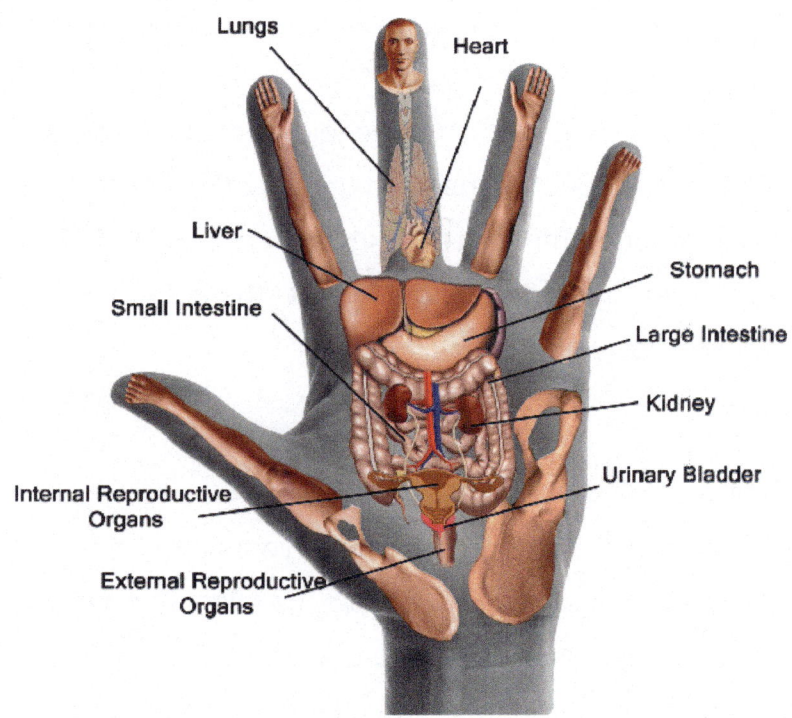

Korean Hand Therapy Correspondence Chart

www.leru-wellness.co.uk

Acupuncture

This is the only therapy here I'm not personally trained in, but I've included it as I know many people have benefitted from it in managing symptoms. Try to find a therapist who is trained in Chinese medicine, not just acupuncture. Then you will also receive advice on herbal teas and supplements and they may use other techniques such as cupping, ear seeds and moxibustion. A Chinese medicine doctor will also look at you holistically, that is they will treat you as a whole person, mind and body in an attempt to get to the root cause of your problem, not just base your treatment on your symptoms.

For those a little worried or needle-phobic please be reassured that acupuncture needles are very fine and only go into the skin around 1mm depth. They are not painful and once in place you shouldn't be able to feel them, they really are nothing to worry about!

Reiki

I've been practising Reiki for over fifteen years and I still cannot describe it in a way which does it justice. Put simply, Reiki is energy and it is all around us. A practitioner will channel that energy through them and into the receiver. I often liken it to putting your phone on charge; if your battery is low, you're maybe not performing your best, giving yourself a charge will boost your levels back up again and get you performing at your optimum. Everyone experiences Reiki differently, some people feel an intense heat, others see colours but almost all find it deeply relaxing. I encourage you to give it a try with an open mind, if it's not for you, then you can move on with the knowledge it's not right for you. And if it is for you, then congratulations! You're one step closer to managing your symptoms!

If you do decide to go down the complementary therapy route, then whichever treatment you choose the most important factor is to choose one you enjoy and with a practitioner whom you feel comfortable with. Most of these treatments 'work' by causing deep relaxation, allowing the brain to reset and release all of those happy hormones we've already discussed. If you are uncomfortable, anxious or simply not enjoying the treatment for any reason, then it will not be as effective.

I am often asked 'How often should I have a treatment?' Whilst there is no easy answer to that, it often depends on time and budget constraints as well as how you feel after a treatment; I do suggest weekly at first, until you see an improvement. Then dropping it to fortnightly and finally, once you've reached your goals then a monthly maintenance session. Just like reactions to medications vary

www.leru-wellness.co.uk

between people, treatments can have different affects on different people. So, if after three sessions you are seeing no improvement, I'd suggest trying another treatment as it maybe the original one isn't right for you.

Essential Oils

Using essential oils for self-care is gaining in popularity and it's easy to see why. Relatively cheap, natural and easily available, they are often touted as a miracle hack for just about everything. If you're new to the world of essential oils, please see the appendix at the back for how to use and safety guidance (even if you have used essential oils before you may still want to check it out since advice varies

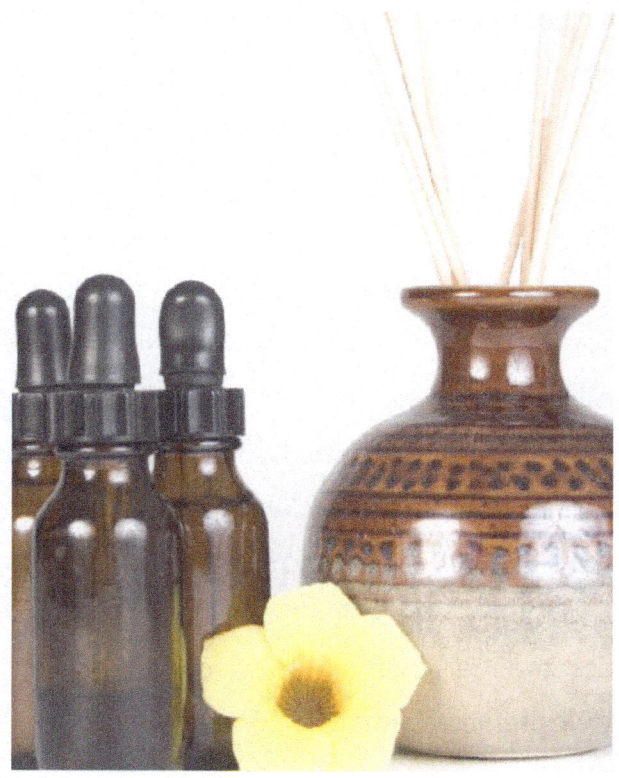

© Sheli Saldana Dreamstime.com

especially between qualified aromatherapists and sales people!).

Essential oils differ from fragrance and perfumery in that they are concentrated extracts from the actual plant material. They therefore contain the healing properties of said plant which may help with a range of symptoms and issues.

There are many products available containing essential oils, especially bath salts and balms which claim to ease pain and exercise related fatigue. By all means try a few and experiment to see if any work for you, just ensure they contain essential oils. Many commercially produced products claim they contain 'lavender' for example, but when examining the ingredients it is actually lavender fragrance and so despite smelling like lavender, will not contain the therapeutic benefits of the oil. As a general rule, you get what you pay for and so if a product is cheap it will likely be fragrance rather than essential oils. Another instance of brands trying to greenwash, is by adding a tiny amount of the essential oil so that they can claim the product contains essential oils, but actually the quantity is such a tiny amount it will have no therapeutic value. Try to stick to 'natural' brands and look on the ingredients label, essential oils will be listed under their botanical name.

It follows therefore, that the only way to know you are getting the full benefit of essential oils is to make your own blends and products, unique to you and suited to your own personal preference. The following are the oils of most benefit to pain and fatigue and also how to best use them.

Top five Essential Oils to ease fatigue

Basil

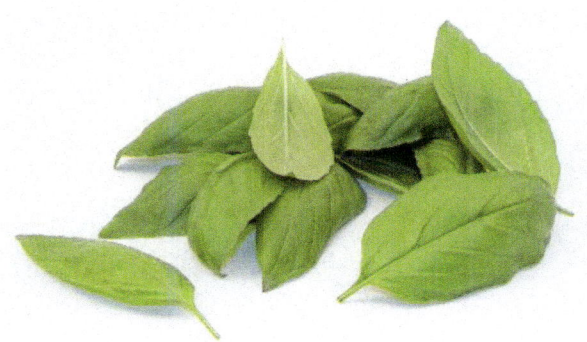

© Deckard73 Dreamstime.com

Extracted from the leaves and flowers, Basil essential oil is considered one of the best oils for the brain. Clearing the head, relieving mental fatigue and giving clarity are all reported, making it ideal for brain fog.

Try to chose 'sweet basil' or European grown varieties. There have been some safety concerns over Asian grown varieties which contain high amounts of the chemical methyl chavicol, linked to liver issues. Although when applied through the skin in the small amounts used in aromatherapy, it is not generally considered an issue, however I'm a believer in erring on the side of caution, especially if you are going to use the oil regularly and when safer alternatives are available.

Lemon

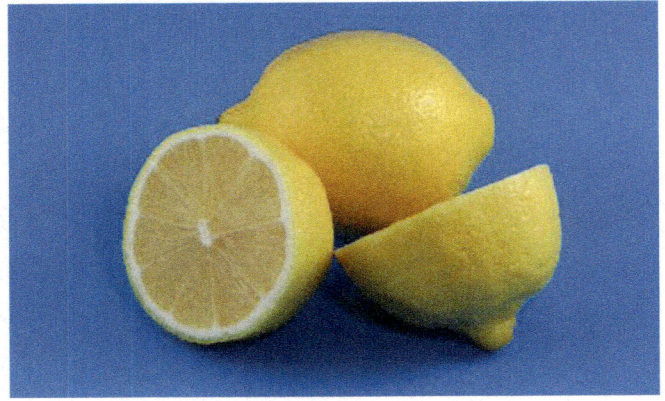

©Ilya Genkin Dreamstime.com

Not only does lemon essential oil help to overcome mental fatigue, it is also excellent for boosting circulation and the lymphatic system. This makes it a good choice on sedentary days.

Be careful going out into the sun after applying to the skin, it is phototoxic meaning it will make your skin burn quicker so stick to the shade.

Rosemary

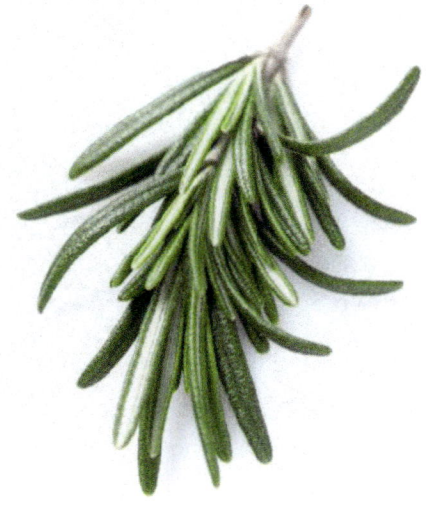

©Anton Ignatenco Dreamstime.com

Another oil excellent for stimulating the brain and nervous system, it has been shown to improve concentration and memory. It is also beneficial if you have low blood pressure and is my go-to oil for headaches and migraines.
Not recommended during pregnancy or if you suffer with epilepsy or have high blood pressure.

www.leru-wellness.co.uk

Cajeput

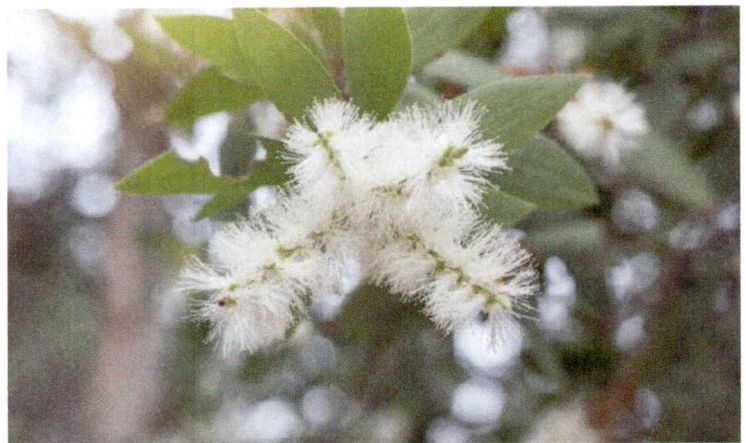

© Pannarai Nak-Im iStock

Stemming originally from Malaysia and Indonesia, Cajeput is another tonic to the nervous system, alleviating fatigue and drowsiness.

Thyme

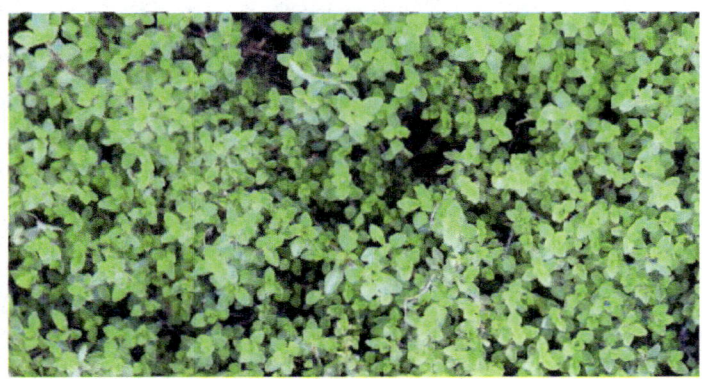

© Oseland Dreamstime.com

Similar to rosemary, thyme oil helps to stimulate the nervous system, improve memory and increase blood pressure. It can also stimulate appetite and circulation.

For some with M.E. rather than generic fatigue, or fibromyalgia these oils may be too stimulating on the nervous system for you. Always start small, one or two oils in small quantities and increase the oils or concentration as you get used to them. Other oils you may wish to consider are Grapefruit, Petitgrain, Bergamot and Lavender. These are all calming oils and will help to balance out an overwrought, stressed nervous system.

For all of these oils, I would advise that the best way to use them is either in a bath or diffused in a room using either an electronic diffuser or one with a tea light. Breathing in the aromas allows the oils to enter the circulatory system and travel to the brain for the best effect.

Fight the fatigue bath oil recipe

- 15ml (around a tablespoon) of unscented bath oil or bubble bath, (most aromatherapy suppliers will sell this as a 'base' product).
- 4 drops Basil
- 4 drops Lemon
- 4 drops Thyme

Mix the essential oils in your chosen base product and disperse under running water. You can also add a handful of epsom salts to the bath water, especially if you have muscle aches.

Using the same ratios you could also add the essential oils to a plain carrier oil and place in a rollerball bottle. Keep the bottle with you incase a bout of fatigue hits, apply to pulse points as and when necessary.

Top five essential oils for pain relief

Black Pepper

A warming oil which promotes circulation, Black Pepper is traditionally used for the majority of pain related conditions; rheumatism, arthritis, muscular aches, stiffness and muscle fatigue. Due to its pain beating flexibility, It is commonly used in sports massage or after exercise to relieve the muscles.

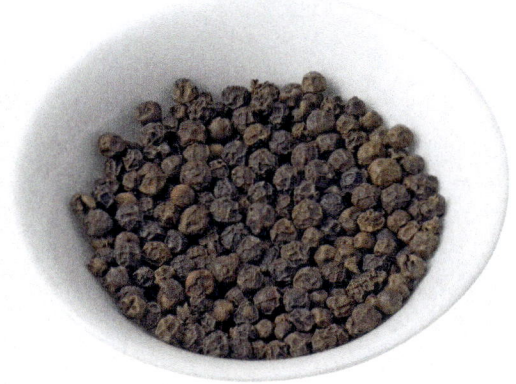

©Alexfiodorov dreamstime.com

www.leru-wellness.co.uk

Sweet Marjoram

Another warming and analgesic oil suitable for any type of muscular strain. It is also useful for the nervous system and so may help with nerve and chronic pain.

A word of warning though, it is reportedly an anaphrodisiac meaning it could lower your sex drive. It can also dull the senses and cause drowsiness so is definitely not an oil to use everyday or if you are already fatigued. It is also best to avoid during pregnancy.

Ginger

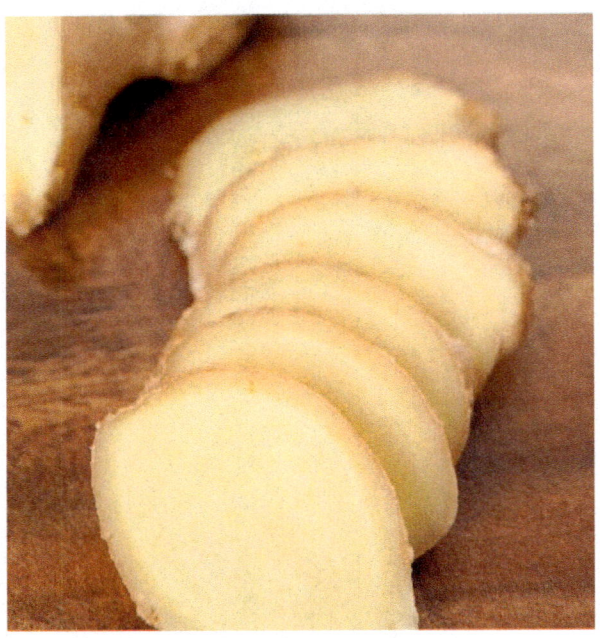

©Rozmarina Dreamstime.com

Ginger is recommended for cold hands and feet as well as muscular and arthritic pain due to its circulation boosting properties.

Peppermint

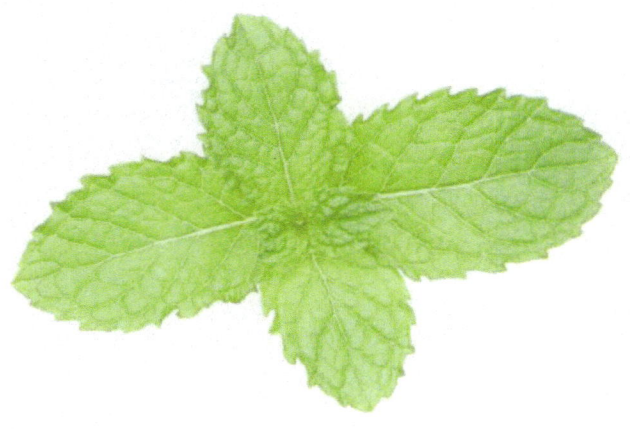

© Winai Tepsuttinun Dreamstime.com

Peppermint has local anaesthetic properties making it ideal for muscular pain. Commonly used in sports massage oil blends for its warming and circulation boosting properties.

www.leru-wellness.co.uk

Pine

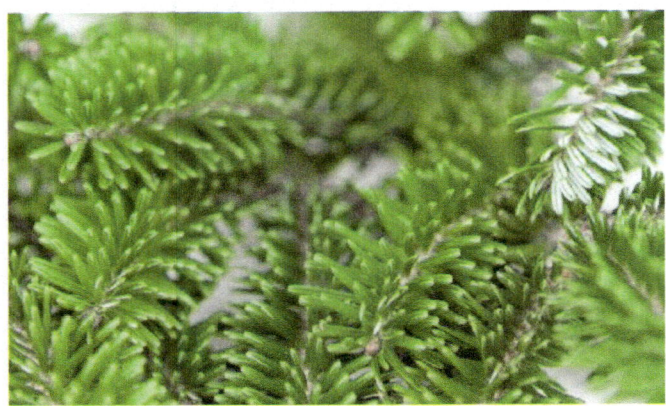

© Wieslaw Fila Dreamstime.com

Pine oil is another oil which stimulates the circulatory system making it useful for relieving pain conditions.

Other oils you may wish to consider as useful pain relieving oils are Frankincense, Sandalwood and Myrrh. Though these are more expensive than the others listed, they help to calm the nervous system and so are more useful for fibromyalgia and similar nervous system pain conditions.

If you are struggling with both pain and fatigue then from the oils already mentioned, rosemary, cajeput, thyme and pine will be the ones most useful for you as they cover both pain and fatigue.

To use any of these oils, add them to a bath (see the fatigue bath oil recipe for quantities) or a plain body cream or balm and apply to the affected area. The oils will then get directly to where they are needed.

Muscle ease balm

- 15ml (a tablespoon) of unscented cream or balm
- 5 drops Black Pepper
- 4 drops Ginger
- 3 drops Peppermint

Mix the oils thoroughly in your base cream, if using a balm you may need to melt it gently in a Bain Marie or microwave first and then allow to cool.

Massage into affected areas up to twice a day.

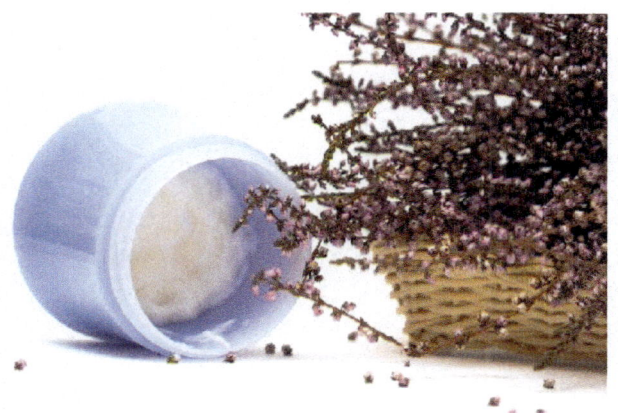

© Viktoriia Kulish Dreamstime.com

Your 'Bad Day' Toolkit

The nature of your condition means everyday changes, sometimes for no apparent reason and so beyond your control. Having a plan in place for such days is not defeatist, it makes practical sense and will hopefully make recovery quicker. Taking a couple of moments to consider what a bad day looks like for you and the steps you can take to make them easier for you, means you will be prepared for when such days arise; and sorry to say they will!

Some issues you may wish to consider;

Work/College

Can you work from home? If not how will you make up your hours? Would a freelance position whereby you work when you feel able be more suitable? Can you realistically continue at your current pace or do you need to consider reducing your hours?

Support Network

Will you need additional help on such days? Particularly around child/pet care and others who may rely on you. Do you feel safe and able to manage on your own? If not who

www.leru-wellness.co.uk

can you rely on to contact for help? What if they are unavailable? Having a strong support network is not only practical, but eases any anxiety you may feel over being unable to manage your responsibilities on such days

Nutrition

Meal prepping is your friend here! I cook in batches and always keep two or three portions in the freezer. If I'm having a day when standing in the kitchen, chopping vegetables is too much effort, then all I need to do is reheat a frozen meal and know I'm still getting a home-cooked, nutritious and unprocessed meal.

Hydration

We've already discussed how important it is to keep hydrated. If going back and forth to the kitchen is too much, then keep flasks of hot drinks and metallic bottles of cold water beside you.

Essential Oils

Keep to hand your diffuser and your go-to oils. If you have pre-prepared a fatigue blend rollerball or pain relief balm, then keep them on your person to use throughout the day.

Activities

We know by now that wallowing in self-pity is not doing us any favours. Keep your mind active and distract yourself from your symptoms with whichever methods work best for you; puzzles, knitting, reading etc. Pop on your favourite movies or music and use the time for some escapism.

Sleep

If you need to sleep then sleep. However be mindful not to knock your natural body clock out by sleeping too much or too late in the day. Doing so will cause you to struggle to get back into your sleep routine and you may have some sleepless nights, furthering your fatigue.

www.leru-wellness.co.uk

Over to You!

It's all well and good reading advice but real change is only achievable when we take action. Use the following pages to discover any triggers, reflect, track your progress and set your goals.

For a PDF version to print or fill in on your device, scan the following QR code.

www.leru-wellness.co.uk

daily PLANNER

MONDAY

TOP PRIORITIES:

_____

_____

TO-DO-LIST:

_____

_____

I'M GRATEFUL FOR: **TODAY'S AFFIRMATION:**

MOOD:
1   2   3   4   5

SLEEP RATING:
1   2   3   4   5

FOOD DIARY: **SYMPTOMS:**

Food Diary	Symptoms
Breakfast	
Lunch	
Dinner	
Snack	

Daily totals: Water   Caffeine   Alcohol   Plant Foods

daily PLANNER

TUESDAY

TOP PRIORITIES:

_____

_____

TO-DO-LIST:

_____

_____

I'M GRATEFUL FOR: **TODAY'S AFFIRMATION:**

MOOD:

1   2   3   4   5

SLEEP RATING:

1   2   3   4   5

FOOD DIARY: **SYMPTOMS:**

Breakfast	
Lunch	
Dinner	
Snack	

Daily totals: Water   Caffeine   Alcohol   Plant Foods

www.leru-wellness.co.uk

daily PLANNER

WEDNESDAY

TOP PRIORITIES:

_____

_____

TO-DO-LIST:

_____

_____

I'M GRATEFUL FOR: **TODAY'S AFFIRMATION:**

MOOD:

1 2 3 4 5

SLEEP RATING:

1 2 3 4 5

FOOD DIARY: **SYMPTOMS:**

Food Diary	Symptoms
Breakfast	
Lunch	
Dinner	
Snack	

Daily totals: Water   Caffeine   Alcohol   Plant Foods

daily PLANNER

THURSDAY

TOP PRIORITIES:

_____

_____

TO-DO-LIST:

_____

_____

I'M GRATEFUL FOR: **TODAY'S AFFIRMATION:**

MOOD:

1 2 3 4 5

SLEEP RATING:

1 2 3 4 5

FOOD DIARY: **SYMPTOMS:**

Breakfast	
Lunch	
Dinner	
Snack	

Daily totals: Water   Caffeine   Alcohol   Plant Foods

www.leru-wellness.co.uk

daily PLANNER

FRIDAY

TOP PRIORITIES:

_____

_____

TO-DO-LIST:

_____

_____

I'M GRATEFUL FOR:

TODAY'S AFFIRMATION:

MOOD:

1 2 3 4 5

SLEEP RATING:

1 2 3 4 5

FOOD DIARY:

SYMPTOMS:

Breakfast	
Lunch	
Dinner	
Snack	

Daily totals: Water   Caffeine   Alcohol   Plant Foods

daily PLANNER

SATURDAY

TOP PRIORITIES:

_____

_____

TO-DO-LIST:

_____

_____

I'M GRATEFUL FOR: **TODAY'S AFFIRMATION:**

MOOD:

1 2 3 4 5

SLEEP RATING:

1 2 3 4 5

FOOD DIARY: **SYMPTOMS:**

Breakfast	
Lunch	
Dinner	
Snack	

Daily totals: Water   Caffeine   Alcohol   Plant Foods

www.leru-wellness.co.uk

daily PLANNER

SUNDAY

TOP PRIORITIES:

_____

_____

TO-DO-LIST:

_____

_____

I'M GRATEFUL FOR: TODAY'S AFFIRMATION:

MOOD:

1   2   3   4   5

SLEEP RATING:

1   2   3   4   5

FOOD DIARY: SYMPTOMS:

FOOD DIARY	SYMPTOMS
Breakfast	
Lunch	
Dinner	
Snack	

Daily totals: Water   Caffeine   Alcohol   Plant Foods

weekly SUCCESS

DATE:

REVIEW YOUR WEEK, AND MAKE SURE TO COMPLETE THE QUESTIONS BELOW IN FULL.

WHAT I HAVE ACHIEVED?

WHAT AM I PROUD OF THIS WEEK?

WHAT HAVE I LEARNED THIS WEEK?

WHAT AM I GRATEFUL THIS WEEK?

WHAT ONE THING COULD I DO DIFFERENTLY NEXT WEEK?

www.leru-wellness.co.uk

goals LIST

WRITE DOWN THE GOALS YOU *REALLY* WANT TO ACHIEVE:
INCLUDE A MIX OF SHORT, MEDIUM AND LONG-TERM GOALS

01

02

03

04

05

06

07

08

goal PLANNER

THE GOAL:

THE STRATEGY:

NEXT ACTIONS:

NOTES:

www.leru-wellness.co.uk

vision BOARD

USE THIS WORKSHEET TO SET GOALS AND PLAN YOUR NEXT YEAR.

I WANT TO STOP:

I WANT TO LEARN:

I WANT TO TRY:

I WANT TO CONTINUTE TO:

I WANT TO BE:

vision PLANNER

PLAN 3 MAIN GOALS YOU HAVE FOR NEXT YEAR. WRITE THEM DOWN AND THE ACTIONS YOU WILL TAKE TO ACHIEVE THEM.

GOAL 1:

GOAL 2:

GOAL 3:

ACTIONS:

_____
_____
_____
_____
_____
_____

ACTIONS:

_____
_____
_____
_____
_____
_____

ACTIONS:

_____
_____
_____
_____
_____
_____

www.leru-wellness.co.uk

30-DAY
Activity Tracker

01	02	03	04	05
06	07	08	09	10
11	12	13	14	15
16	17	18	19	20
21	22	23	24	25
26	27	28	29	30

Aromatherapy and Essential Oil Safety advice

There has been a huge increase in the use of essential oils in recent years. This is partly due to well-meaning bloggers and social media claiming cheap and effective cures for any ailment. However with that, has come a myriad of sales lies, dangerous misinformation and even hospitalisations due to misuse. As a professional and qualified Aromatherapist, I feel it is my duty to include the following guidelines when advising people to use essential oils at home. If you are in any doubt however, please seek advice from a qualified aromatherapist, we undertake thorough training in the safety aspect of using essential oils and it is in our interest to raise the standard and respect of the aromatherapy industry. Retailers however, have received little to no training and are often only interested in making a sale!

Firstly when it comes to buying oils, always chose a respectable retailer. There are several online but my personal favourites are 'Naturally Thinking' or 'Base Formula'. Both sell good quality essential oils and associated products at a reasonable price. Beware of oils which seem cheap, they are often fragrance oils i.e. they smell the same as the oil but do not have the therapeutic qualities of an essential oil, or have already been diluted down. Oils should usually come in a dark, glass bottle and have a dropper. These are all to preserve the oil for as long as possible. Oils do have a shelf-life, although usually not considered harmful, they may not smell their best or lose some of their therapeutic value. If an oil is thicker, smells different or if crystals are forming around the thread of the bottle top, then consider replacing that oil. Oils should ideally be stored in a cool, dark place e.g. in a cupboard and never in direct sunlight as this speeds up the degradation process.

There is so much more to essential oils than just smelling good. They are extracted from plants and as such are concentrated, complex chemicals. Therefore essential oils should never be used undiluted directly on the skin nor should they be taken internally i.e. added to a pill or worse diluted in water to drink. I often see or hear comments such as 'but if the oil is pure/organic then what is the harm?' The issue is not the purity of the oil, but the fact that as we have previously stated, essential oils are complex, concentrated, chemical compounds. Repeated exposure can cause sensitivities such as rashes and blisters. Plus oil and water do not mix, adding oil to water and then drinking it still means undiluted oil can come into contact with your stomach lining causing internal blisters and ulcers. Some oils can also cause organ damage when taken internally, this has even resulted in death. Put simply ingesting oils is not worth the risk!

With regards to the 'organic' label; essential oils fall under cosmetics rather than food or pharmaceuticals. Therefore the terms 'pure' and 'organic' mean nothing, there is no legislation protecting these terms when used in cosmetics, meaning any cosmetic can claim to be 'organic'. These terms are simply a marketing ploy, if you really want to check a cosmetic/essential oil is organic then seek out ones which carry the Soil Association logo. Whilst essential oils made from organically grown plants may have environmental benefits, the jury is still out as to whether the oil itself has a better therapeutic value and therefore standard safety advice still applies.

Some essential oils are not suitable for people with certain medical conditions, including pregnancy, high blood pressure or when taking medications so please check each oil you intend to use. Also extra caution needs to be taken when using oils with children, several should be avoided and dilutions are higher. Guidelines constantly change around this issue and since this guide in intended for adults, seek the latest advise if you wish to use oils on children. Some animals also metabolise essential oils differently to humans, resulting in adverse effects. Please check when using essential oils in a diffuser around pets. The topic is too exhaustive for this guide but a main example is not to expose dogs to Tea Tree oil.

www.leru-wellness.co.uk

Some oils are also more prone to cause sensitisation in people e.g. cause rashes due to overuse. This is why it is advised to use oils sparingly (remember less is more!) and to not keep using the same oils repeatedly.

Essential Oils - How To Use

Probably the most common way to use essential oils at home is using a diffuser; either one with a tea light or an electric steam diffuser. Personally I prefer a steam diffuser as they do not use heat which can degrade the oil, meaning the oil smells stronger. Always follow manufacturers instructions but for either diffusers usually 5-6 drops of oil added to water is all that is needed to fill your room with fragrance.

If you wish to use oils on your skin, remember they need to be diluted, usually to around 2% value (i.e. 2ml of total essential oil in 98ml of base product) Aromatherapy suppliers have a whole range of base products you can add oils to including carrier oils, creams, shampoos and shower gels.

If using in a bath, please remember water and oil do not mix! Your oils still need diluting in a base bath product and then adding to the water. Without such, the essential oil will float on the surface of the water and come into contact with your skin on getting in the bath. I see many well-meaning recipes online advising people to mix oils with bath salts, however they do not mix very well either. By all means throw in a handful of epsom/Himalayan salts into your bath but add your essential oils in a suitable base separately.

Thank You!

My motivation in my work, both in the treatment room and in writing these guides has always been to improve the health and therefore lives of my clients. I truly hope you have found some of the suggestions in this book useful and are beginning to reap the benefits.

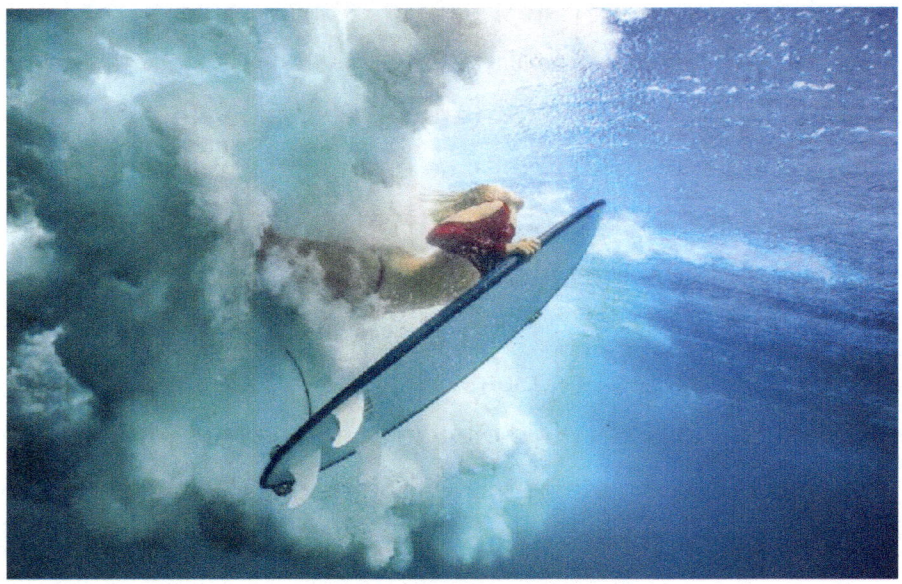

© WillyamBradberry Dreamstime.com

I'd love to know how you are getting on, so do keep in touch via my Instagram @leruwellness or join my mailing list and receive a free e-guide to using essential oils around the home by clicking on the following qr code

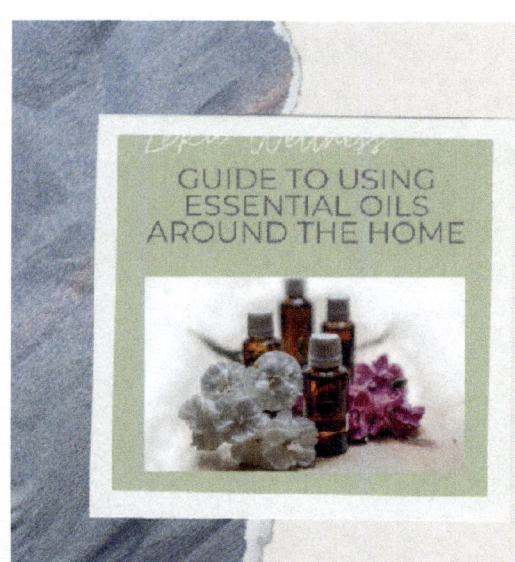

JOIN MY MAILING LIST

Be the first to hear about new titles

As an independent author, reviews are so important in helping spread the word and giving credibility to my work. So, if you have a spare minute, I'd be really grateful if you could leave me a review on Amazon.

www.leru-wellness.co.uk

Resources

britishpainsociety.org

meassociation.org.uk

www.fmauk.org

www.bant.org.uk

www.wimhofmethod.com

iquitsugar.com

[1] Phillippa Lally et al. How are habits formed: Modelling habit formation in the real world. *Eur J Soc*. **40**, 998-1009 (2010)

[2] medicalnewstoday.com - Does Sugar Cause Inflammation in the Body?

[3] Carlton and Orr. The effects of fluid loss on physical performance: A critical review. *J Sport and Health Science*. **4**, 357-363 (2015)

[4] The Washington Post - Can Tart Cherries Help Reduce Inflammation and Pain? 23/2/24

[5] nah.gov - Studies Find Microbiome Changes may be a Signature for ME/CFS 8/2/23

[6] Metin and Ozdemir. The Effects or Aromatherapy Massage and Reflexology on Pain and Fatigue in Patients with Rheumatoid Arthritis: A Randomized Controlled Trial. *Pain Management Nursing.* **17 Issue 2,** 140-149 (2016)
Gunnarsdottir and Peden-McAlpine. Effects of Reflexology on Fibromyalgia Symptoms: A multiple case-study. *Comp. Therapies in Clinical Practice.* **16 Issue 3,** 167-172 (2010)

www.leru-wellness.co.uk

Printed in Great Britain
by Amazon